To eat in silence, is to truly hear.

~ Ramona Brown

My Qualifications as a weight loss expert

What qualifies me to write this book? I have gained and lost thousands of pounds and ate tons of food. That is what qualifies me. If you want to know about saturated fats, carbohydrates versus calories, triglycerides, cholesterol, or how sugar is metabolized and what your pancreas does, this is not the book for you. I am not a medical doctor. You should consult your physician before beginning any weight loss program. That's why he or she makes the big bucks.

My Background

First let me tell you a little bit about myself. I did weigh 280 lbs. I say "did" cause right now after 3 days I weigh 264 pounds. I have basically been fat all my life. As a child my nickname was "baby blimp" a name given to me because there was a popular wrestler at the time in the 1960's which wore a diaper. I suppose I looked like him. The nickname was later adjusted to "Blimp" and finally dropped all together when I entered elementary school. I was the youngest of three children, born to two people who never finished high school. I will spare you the, "We were so poor speech." We did have some funny jokes about that. We use to say we were poor with 3 O's and we were so poor we thought, "Not to be sold or exchanged" was a brand name. We were so poor the burglar broke into our home and all he got was practice.

I didn't get to 280 pounds overnight. I am 49 years old and it has been a rough journey. Eating for all the wrong reasons.

Many times as a child I would go to look in the refrigerator and find only butter and ketchup. I think this scarcity of food later led to me actually "hoarding" food in my house and also oddly enough in my body. On the plus side we weren't raised on a lot of junk food or sugary cereals. As a child I ate mostly brown beans, fried potatoes, cornbread and wild game. Not the best diet but not the worse either. Too much salt and grease for sure.

Looking back I realize now my mother was more than likely anorexic, at least according to the old Polaroid's that captured the image of her bony hips in a sky blue pantsuit with her beehive hairdo. That's okay though, she didn't have to eat because I was eating enough for both of us, she made sure of that. Practically force-feeding me. Oh did I mention she was the lunch lady at our school. I always got extra helpings.

During first through sixth grades I would not say I was fat. I was actually tall for my age in 4th grade but everyone eventually caught up to me and passed me concerning height. I reached 5'2" in Eighth grade and never got any taller. That's right, I am 5'2" and 264lbs. That is morbidly obese. A BMI of 18.5 is considered underweight, 18.5-24.9 is considered normal weight. 25.0 – 29.9 is considered overweight. 30-34.9 is considered class I obesity. 35-39.9 is class II obesity. Over 40 is considered class III obesity. My BMI was 51.2, very scary.

How I became a binge eater

I don't remember when I began binge eating. I remember coming home from school and frying a whole skillet of homemade French fries and eating the whole pan full. I remember waiting until everyone left and eating biscuits dipped in mayonnaise. I know, that is terribly gross and I hate sharing such personal information but my goal is to help other people who have the same problem as I did. I was hungry all the time. I was hungry and I could not stop being hungry no matter how much I ate or what I ate.

Crazy diets that didn't help

At times I would try to lose weight. Once I lost 80 pounds on a popular diet program. How I suffered? I thought about food constantly. The diet had me fixing these low calorie recipes. I swear I spent half the day in the kitchen prepping something only I could eat and the other half cooking for everyone else. What good is being skinny if you never get out of the kitchen? Another diet was "Two shakes and a sensible dinner." If I had any earthly idea what a sensible dinner meant I would not have been at 280 pounds. Actually that diet turned out to be a really healthy way to gain weight. I would still binge eat and I still drank the two shakes so I got plenty of vitamins and iron along with way too many calories.

I tried another diet where you drank this liquid powdered cement stuff, and ate only meat. You had to check your pee to see if the little test strip turned blue. I still don't know what that was about. That diet made me really cranky, my family insisted I quit that one.   We would weigh in groups and once I lost the most weight that week and they gave me a "No-belly prize." I was totally humiliated and never went back.

What weight I did lose I kept it off for about 15 minutes and before you know it I had gained that back and even more.

I laugh when people say, "You have to have willpower." Because nothing is further from the truth. Willpower has absolutely nothing to do with losing weight. No one has had more willpower than I have. Most overweight people I know are the strongest willed, intelligent, people you will ever meet. When skinny people say, "You just have to watch what you eat." I can bust out laughing now. Because they have no idea what they are talking about. I know the secret to losing weight and it has absolutely nothing to do with any of that. I have had many observations about weight loss. I have heard skinny women say, "How can they not control their food?" I have been in fast food restaurants and seen skinny women order cheeseburger fries, milkshake while I order a salad, yet they are skinny and I am fat. Why?

The reason I am fat is because I binge eat. Once while the family was sitting with a sick relative at the hospital I saw a friend eat a half of a sandwich and a cup of coffee, and when someone offered her something else to eat she said, "No thanks I'm full." I remember thinking, "Are you serious?"

What I ate on binge, you would be amazed

I use to eat 4 or 5 sandwiches at a time. I use to eat 4 or 5 "Jethro Bowls" of cereal. I would eat a half pot of soup, and these weren't the times I was on a binge. Once on a binge I ate an entire large bag of jumbo corn chips with a whole can bean dip an entire box of snack cakes and a large milk shake. What can I say? I didn't die from that, which is surprising, I didn't even throw up. Before I was married with children I would often pull up to drive thru fast food restaurants and order massive amounts of food. Those were my favorite. I could secretly pull off into a deserted area of the parking lot and eat in peace, without having to submit to the stares from strangers. It was nothing for me to make four or five trips to an all you eat buffet.

I did not binge and purge, I just binged. These were not my proudest moments but now I know it was also not my fault.

It is not easy to be a binge eater. It takes careful planning. You have to have alone time. If you live alone it is no problem, but if you have a family it takes special planning. Many nights I would stay home when my husband went out with friends, I would stay home to continue my love affair with food. Sometimes I would stay up late and eat after everyone else had gone to bed. Now I know this was not emotional eating. I was physically hungry. If you can imagine being hungry ALL the time. That was my life.

Dieting meant suffering. Pacing back and forth in the kitchen. I would open and shut the refrigerator a thousand times.

I know my family felt sorry for me. Sometimes they would encourage me to just eat. They didn't understand, one bite meant an hour long binge until I was miserable, sick and guilty. I wouldn't even remember all I ate. I went into the "Zone" and just ate and ate.

Being 280 pounds and five feet two inches tall comes with its own set of problems. While trying to exercise I injured my knee. It is still very painful, I had one surgery on it but now it is inoperable. I developed Type II Diabetes. You would think that would be enough to scare me into losing weight. No matter how hard I tried I could not go without eating. I had people tell me I needed to lose weight. Friends, family, and doctors. Really? Do you think? As if I may not have realized it.

The Quiet Diet Discovery:

Now let me tell you about how we found out the solution to weight gain. One evening we were all sitting around eating dinner. We live in a very small house and there are three of us that live here. My son was also visiting. We were eating in the living room.   Which I know people are going to say that is bad but our house is so small it is not like we have a huge dining room. Anyway we are sitting around eating and my son begins to tell us about how sensitive he is to sound. He has always had a hypersensitivity to sound and light. He is 21 and we already knew he was sensitive to it. Once when he was eleven years old I had to rush him home from a carnival. We live in a small town and the carnival only comes through once a year. He had been looking forward to it and saving his money. Finally the evening came and we packed up and headed to the carnival. After about 30 minutes he found me waiting in line with his sister and pleaded with me to take him home. The flashing lights and noises from the carnival were just too much for him to bare.

Another incident occurred when he turned 18 years old. In our area there are not many jobs. My son is Native American and quite a few of his peers had been hired at a nearby casino. We decided to drive up and let him look around to see if this might be a place he would like to work. By this time I had forgotten about the carnival incident. Well you can imagine the effect of all those bells, whistles and lights at the slot machines had on him. He was ready to leave as soon as we got there. He is happily employed now for three years in a quieter atmosphere. However his sensitivity to sound, although annoying to him, turned out to be my saving grace.

My son was struggling to tell us over dinner that he could hear how loud we were eating and it was really getting on his nerves. He said he could hear us smacking and slurping and it drove him crazy. He also added that on the very few times we had went out to eat together that he found it embarrassing that we all ate so loud.

I never considered myself a loud eater. I always chew my food with my mouth closed. I guess I never really thought about it at all. He told me, "You eat really loud," and then he said the magic words, "You should hear yourself."

I have always had a little bit of a hearing problem. I talk louder than most people probably because I can't hear as well. I decided to plug up my ear and see if I could hear myself chewing. So I did. Wow, that's weird I thought. I can hear every slurp, every bite, and every swallow. I ate the rest of my meal that way, just to listen. What can I say, it's a small town and we are hard up for entertainment here.

A funny thing happened when I had finished eating I had only eaten the contents of one bowl but I was stuffed beyond belief. I could not eat another bite. At first I thought something was wrong, like maybe the food was gassy or something. Why did I fill up so fast? I started talking about it with the family. My daughter who is the scientist in the family made an observation. "Mom that is why you eat so much, your brain doesn't realize you are full." She had been taking anatomy and physiology classes at high school and explained to me that they tell fat people to chew slowly, eat on a smaller plate, wait 20 minutes after you eat to let your brain know that you are full blah blah blah. I had always read those kinds of useless tips in women's magazines. Of course none of those things ever worked for me. My brain had no earthly idea how to stop eating.

It dawned on me this is some kind of physical medical problem. My binge eating is not emotional. You have heard that fat people eat to bury their feelings. That is not true. Fat people eat because they do not have that switch in their head to tell them they are full. Fat people are different from skinny people. You don't have to count calories, points, exercise etc. to lose weight. As soon as you expend more calories then you take in, you will lose weight. In order to maintain a weight of 280 pounds you have to take in a lot of calories.

I began to stop up my ears with earplugs every time I ate. It was a miracle. I began to journal to keep some sort of record of my weight loss and hunger. I dusted off my cheap scales and dug out my diabetes monitor.

Could it be this simple? I began taking pictures each day of my scales and taking my blood sugar.

The first day I weighed after I began my program was Monday Feb. 21, 2011 I weighed 278 pounds.

I had 2 small bowls of soup and one baked apple with raisins and walnuts. I wasn't hungry and I was amazed. Could it be this simple? This must be like what it feels to be normal. Before I was hungry ALL the time. I ate constantly. Imagine eating and eating and never getting full. That is what it feels like to be obese.

At the end of the day I felt a little nausea I don't know why. I hadn't ingested anything. I wonder if it is because I had taken blood pressure, diabetes and joint medicine. It never made me sick before but I don't know. Maybe just drastically cutting my calories made my body pissed off.

After the end of the first day my sugar level was 167.

Tuesday, Feb. 22, 2011 Day 2

268 pounds, Wow, I lost 10 pounds overnight. I remember thinking "Can that even be right?" I have been spending a lot of time in the bathroom. I hadn't been hungry at all. After eating just a small amount I was way past full. Something about my brain, which is hearing every slurp, crunch, and swallow is convincing my brain that I was fuller, faster and with less. I ate one bowl of cereal and a piece of toast; I cut an apple in half and had intended on eating it but couldn't. For lunch I had a chef's salad with ham, cheese and egg with Tuscan dressing it was good and lavish but I could only eat one small bowl. For supper I made myself a stir-fry with sausage, broccoli, bell pepper, green onion and carrots, it was lavish also but again I could only eat one small bowl and gave the rest to my husband. He is also overweight but still skeptical of the plan. My sugar this morning before breakfast, and diabetes

meds was 158.

Wednesday, Feb. 23, 2011 Day 3

264 pounds, I had lost 4 more pounds. This is friggin' amazing. I want to tell everyone about it but my family won't let me. They believe it is our gateway out of poverty. A cure for obesity. I did a search on the Internet and no one is using this method. During a conversation with my son, he remarked that he cannot eat because he thinks his brain can hear people eating and it is tricking his stomach into thinking it is full so he has a distain to eat. He is very skinny and has to make himself eat. Could this also be a cure for anorexia? Could this save people's lives? More study is needed. My sugar is 152 this morning without medicine and before breakfast. For breakfast I had a tuna sandwich and 3 gherkin pickles. My daughter told me to eat whatever I want and not to diet, because if I try to diet I will

lose weight but won't know if it is because of "the program" but if I eat whatever I want and still lose weight then I will know we are on to something.

I began noticing as my husband eats that I could hear him smacking, slurping and swallowing. Oddly enough it made my mouth water. What does that mean? I had to leave the room.

Today for the first time in a year I put my shoes and socks on by myself without assistance. I continue to amaze myself.

I made a doctor's. appointment. In two weeks to see if he can tell if I lost any weight. My husband went to the store and bought me real earplugs cause the paper tissues, that I was using were laying around everywhere.

I asked my son what we should do, like if we should go and tell anyone about this yet and he said we should wait at least a year. Then I said what if someone else comes out with it first and he said you mean how like two people a million miles away from each other come up with the same idea at the same time, like it goes through the air waves or something? He suggested we wrap our heads in tinfoil. That made me laugh at loud. He is like that, so funny. We laughed and laughed.

I should tell you some rules, you can eat anything you want as much as you want, the secret is you "won't want." You cannot eat in front of the TV or eat where there is any noise. You must eat your meal in total silence. No talking you must be able to hear every slurp and swallow.

I had chili pie with cheese, and I just ate one bowl. I think I could have eaten more but I didn't. I didn't feel too deprived as I am full, but I will say I liked it more than other dishes I have eaten in the last three days.

I am convinced the key to losing weight is to focus and to shut the brain off like a light switch when the stomach is full. The brain only recognizes the stomach is full when it can hear yourself slurping, chewing, swallowing, sometimes it helps to close your eyes, while you wear the earplugs. It is very gross to hear yourself chew.

At this point I feel I should add a warning about earplugs, which are the key to this program. I would hope that people would have the common sense to not shove the earplug down into their ear canal. Yes it is possible to get an ear infection. Again, I am not a doctor but myself I would think it is better to have a sore ear than be obese.

In my research I have found: As far as the health of your ear goes studies show that long-term use of foam earplugs can cause ear wax to build up or become impacted. Ear plugs block the outward flow of ear wax that our bodies naturally produce in order to self-clean the ears.

Foam plugs are often pushed in too far, which can also pack the wax deep inside your ear canal, and possibly against the eardrum. You'll end up with constant ringing of the ears (tinnitus), pain, or hearing loss. What's more — not to gross you out — bacteria thrive on warm, moist, foam earplugs, and since they can't be thoroughly cleaned, people often end up with ear infections.

If you can't rest soundly with a closed window, and earplugs are your way to sleep, it's recommended to invest in a custom molded pair

Wow there is a lot to learn about all this. I certainly do not want to hurt anyone or end up in an ugly lawsuit, the earplugs would have to be specially made to be used everyday 3 times or more a day.

What if this is true and right, what if it is a cure for obesity and anorexia as I think it is, and what if people die in the meantime while I am waiting to see if it works, but I can't say something is true without proving it first.

All I had to eat today was two chili pies and a tuna fish sandwich.

Feb. 24, 2011, Day 4

I lost 8 lbs last night I am down to 256, I didn't even wake up hungry. I'm not sure how this diet should work, am I supposed to eat if I am not hungry? I wish I had an expert to ask but in this situation I guess I am the expert. I suppose all of that will come out over time. I haven't weighed 256 in a long time. My sister is shocked and amazed I know she will not believe me when I tell her I lost 8 pounds overnight but I knew I would lose weight fast. I don't know how many calories I was taking in to maintain a weight of 280 probably five or 6000 a day and when I dropped it down to normal-I mean there is just no way to maintain that weight which is good, but the numbers make it sound unbelievable. I got into some jeans that I haven't been in awhile. My sugar is again 152, I guess that is okay that it didn't change. I was reading last night about insulin levels and how that affects hunger and I didn't understand any of it but today I am working on forgiving myself. For so many years I binged and there was so much guilt involved and now I feel like none of that was my fault cause I didn't know any better. I always thought something was wrong with me like I had some kind of mental illness or something.

My teenage daughter was not too happy with me. She had become accustom to this mom that is overweight, kind of a doormat that eats all the time and cooks all the time. I don't think I can be that kind of person anymore. Steve said jokingly, "What if guys start to look at you." I didn't say it but my weight did not keep men from liking me. Certain men, yes but not all men like skinny minnies.

I made myself laugh this morning because I thought, "Wow am I a genius or am I insane? Am I really losing weight and have we really figured out the way to lose weight, can it be this simple? I don't want to tell anyone about it until I have proof. If there is no proof then I am crazy but if there is proof, well honestly we are not really genius's we are just lucky cause we happenstance on to this. I'm giggly. Maybe that is a side effect of the rapid weight loss, I wonder if there is side effects from rapid weight loss, I should look that up.

Side Effects of Rapid Weight Loss

1. While most side effects may be temporary, one of the most severe problems arising out of rapid weight loss is Gallstones. If you suddenly stop eating, there may be a shift in the balance of bile salts and cholesterol. This may turn out to be a lethal concoction for the body. The cholesterol will then form lumps, called gallstones. Gallstones lodge themselves in the bile ducts and can be extremely painful. In some situations, it may also result in inflammation in the liver, pancreas and bladder. Sudden reduction in eating also reduces contractions in the gall bladder, which aids the process of gallstone creation.

2. Another rapid weight loss side effect is loss of muscle mass. If the body does not get the necessary food to fuel its daily activities, it's going to turn to other sources for energy. And ironically, research suggests that it will not use up the fat reserve as the body is programmed to use fat

reserves as the last resort. So, before eating up the fat reserve, your body will first consume the muscle mass.

3. Loss of muscle tissue will lead to loss of water content in the body. The muscle mass comes from protein, which has a significant amount of water. Muscles also store most of the water, so loss of muscle from the body will lead to loss of muscle mass.

4. Another rapid weight loss side effect is hair loss. Hair needs protein for its growth. In fact, hair itself is made of a protein known as keratin. Hence if you decide to go off food, your protein consumption will reduce and there will be no protein available for hair growth, as the body will try to optimize whatever protein it gets. So hair basically pulls out the short straw and is left as the last in the hierarchy functions that protein needs to perform.

5. Other weight loss side effects include shivering. This side effect is temporary and occurs if you have resorted to weight loss surgery. Weight loss surgery dramatically cuts out all the fat from the body. Fat insulates the body and stops the loss of body heat. Once all the fat is lost, the body heat will be lost quickly, leading to shivering.

6. One of the most unsightly side effects of rapid weight loss is hanging skin. When you lose weight, the skin, stretched due the fat, takes some time to tighten itself around the body. In some cases, especially ones related to obese people, there have been instances where people have lost weight too quickly, but their skin still hangs loose because it wasn't given enough time to adapt and wrap itself around the body tightly enough again.

7. And lastly about the dangers of diet pills. Some people consume rapid weight loss pills without being aware of the side effects of weight loss pills. Consuming diet pills may lead to various medical complications such as increasing your heart rate and causing palpitations.

These were the rapid weight loss side effects. While losing weight may be important from the point of view of fitness, you have to remember to do it step by step. Losing weight too fast can bring on the above problems.

Side effects from the Quiet Diet

I have had the shivering, so far no hair loss but I will be watching for that and I probably should be drinking more water. As far as being flabby, trust me that won't bother me, I would much rather be flabby than fat. You can hide flabby, you can't hide fat. I already had my gallbladder out from when I had gallstones when I lost the 80 pounds in my twenties, so I am not sure how that will work. So far the only side effect I have had from the diet is weight loss.

Friday Feb. 25, 2011 Day, 5

Weight 264 Sugar at 165 before Breakfast.

So I am asking myself why I gained the weight and does that mean the program doesn't work? I still believe in the program and I will tell you why. First of all, we all agreed on the program that I could eat anything that I wanted, which is true, it has to be true because that is the only way you can stay on the program long term. So yesterday for breakfast I ate a tuna fish sandwich, for lunch I had chili again and yesterday afternoon I laid down to take a nap at about 3:30 p.m. This is my normal habit but since I had been on the program I had not needed the nap because I had so much energy. I still did not "need' the nap but my son was asleep and so was my husband and there was nothing to do so I laid down. I woke up at about 8 p.m. and although I WAS NOT hungry I decided I should eat anyway because I keep telling myself I need 3 meals. I am a diabetic and don't know how it would affect my health if I quit eating all together but at this point I actually feel like I could not eat at all and I wouldn't be hungry. So last night, after I got up and my son woke up and I decided to cook so I made a stir fry with rice, broccoli, carrots, sausage, onion, bell pepper, soy sauce and a pre-prepared seasoning. I believe I gained weight because of the salt and because of eating so late. I know I could actually skip my evening meal and lose weight but the whole idea of the program is to see if the invention works.

Not everyone wants to see you skinny

Okay this is a good time to talk about people

trying to sabotage your diet. Before when I went on a diet my well meaning husband no matter how many times I told him I needed to lose weight would bring home chips, candy, etc. He had been making some really delicious food. Last night he made a giant plate of French fries which is the one thing I could never resist but now that is like 'no problem" anyway it is like he is doing this subconsciously because I know he would never really want to hurt me. So this morning I am eating. For breakfast I had one slice of bacon, one fried egg and one piece of toast. Now I realize this is not a dieters breakfast but again the deal was I get to eat whatever I want. So while I am eating my breakfast, he turns up the TV in his room full blast so I can't even hear myself think let alone hear myself eat. Then he comes in here and while I am sitting quietly in front of the TV set, he turns the TV set on and full blast then takes my bowl away from me while I am still eating. Now granted my bowl was empty but I still had a piece of bacon in my hand. So this morning we had a family meeting about how important it is for mom to have peace and quiet while she is eating, (which everyone took way to personal) and now everyone is acting like his or her feelings are hurt.

Okay let me say this, I have been on crazy diets before, and of course many didn't work, but I am not asking my family to sacrifice a lot. I am not buying weird foods; I am not asking people to cook for me. I am not leaving my home and staying at the gym all day. I am only asking for peace and quiet during meal times so that I can eat alone. This will not work if you live with a noisy family. You have to have peace, quiet and sometimes you have to close your eyes so you can hear yourself chew better. I really don't think that is a lot to ask.

I hate to call my sister and tell her I gained 3 pounds but I still believe in the program so it's all cool. On a sad note during my research I watched several TV news programs about people having weight loss surgery. I cried, I mean I sincerely really cried because all of that is so unnecessary and it is so much pain to go through, and I wish I could just tell them but I know no one would believe me and maybe I would do more harm than good. Another show upset me, it was about taking fat people and putting them through this tough regime to have them lose weight. There was a lot of yelling and very mean spirited talking to the fat people by skinny people. I really believe this is unnecessary. Why on earth would anyone put up with that?

My advice if you feel like you want to exercise is to find an activity you enjoy doing, such as tennis, bike riding, hiking preferably an activity where no one is yelling.

I can't lie I do want to make money from this, not for me but for my family, and I think of all the people I could help with other things.   If I sell some books the first thing I am going to buy is some towels and something for my family. So yea I would like to make some money but it troubles me that I know in my heart I have the answer and no one will believe me without the data, and people might die from obesity in the meantime.

Later on the same day:

So for lunch I had pork chop, broccoli and green beans. I am still not hungry and this whole idea is driving me crazy. My family is driving me crazy cause I know they are sick of me talking about it.

Feb. 26, 2011

Weight 263, sugar is 196 before meds. Yesterday I had one bacon, one egg, one toast, lunch was a small pork chop, with broccoli and green beans and for supper I had one hot dog on one piece of bread with mustard and relish, but my husband popped pop corn and I ate way too much of that work up at 2 a.m. sick from the popcorn but took 2 antacids. I have no idea how come my sugar is so high.

For breakfast I had a bowl of oat cereal but I fixed my bowl too full and had to empty some of it out and give it to the dog cause there was too much in there. Its like that old saying my eyes are bigger than my stomach. I feel like I have had my stomach stapled. You know I have heard people say that have had that operation that the can just barely eat or they will get sick. I haven't eaten so much that I have gotten sick but I could see how that could happen. The other thing that I would like to warn against is that you really have no desire to eat so I don't know how long you could go without eating without getting sick or hurting yourself. Again I am making myself eat 3 meals a day, but I actually don't even feel like I need to eat at all. Except for the indigestion from the popcorn I haven't had any stomach problems no constipation or diarrhea. I just finished eating bean soup, cornbread and red velvet chocolate birthday cake. (It was my daughter's birthday cake.) The liquid seems to fill me up more than solid foods. I can no longer drink a full can of pop. Sometimes I can only drink from a couple of sips to a half can. I always drink diet pop.

For supper I had roast beef, lettuce and four baby carrots. I was so full I was about to bust, the food tasted so good, but when I was done, I was done and did not want more.

Feb. 27, 2011

Weight 261, sugar 147 before eating or meds. Oh man it feels good to get up and weigh and know that you lost a little weight. Tomorrow it will be exactly one week and so far I have lost 19 pounds. Food tastes so good now to. I like crunchy things. My portion sizes are extremely small but every time I eat I feel like I have over ate. Life is good. Things are normal. This is the life I should have been living all along, a life where food is no longer the MOST important thing in my life. Food is now just something you stop and eat every once in awhile. I emailed several doctors yesterday well two, to be exact one at a famous clinic and one from Tulsa that is doing a diabetes study. I am sure I sounded like a crazy woman. I am just so excited but everyone in my family keeps telling me. You have to be tested, have data before you can prove what you say. I feel like I am in the twilight zone sometimes.

Later in the day: My knees hurt. The extra energy I have from losing the 19 pounds is causing me to be up on my feet too long and making my knees hurt. I sent an email to the clinic about my idea. I don't know if they will respond I am sure they think I am crazy I had 3 meals today, oatmeal, oriental, and taco salad for supper but about 8:30 I had an irresistible craving for a small glass of tomato juice. I ended up drinking 2 small glasses. I do not know what that means. I hope it doesn't ruin my progress.

Feb. 28, 2011

  Weight 256 Sugar 151 if ever there was a day to overeat it would be today but so far I haven't. I did get really stressed out. This is a small town and I heard an untrue bit of gossip about myself. I barely had time to eat. This morning I had a bologna sandwich, for breakfast I had a cup of ramen and for lunch I am going to see if I can get my husband to make me a hamburger slider with grilled onions. I wore some jeans today that I hadn't been able to get into in years. That is awesome. 24 pounds in one week, no one will ever believe this, (until I lose some more weight) I sent several emails to the clinic and several doctors but I was right no one is going to believe me. I asked myself how would I react if someone had told me this was the cure for obesity. Of course I would think they were crazy.

March 1, 2011

Weight 251 sugar 136 Today was my day to go to the school to get news for the newsletter. I thought for sure someone would say I looked like I had lost weight but no such luck. One of my friends almost did. She said, 'Wow you look good today." And I said, "Yea I feel really feel good today," and she said, "Any special reason are you doing anything different?" (She knows I struggle with joint pain and I wasn't for sure if she was saying I looked thinner or if she meant I didn't look like I was in pain.) So I said, "Well you know, I have good days and bad days and today is a good day." I went over to the man I consider my boss and talked to him and he said, "Sit down and eat with us." Everyone at the table was having pizza and I noticed he was having a small salad. I said, "I actually already ate." And he said, "What did you have and I said, "I had a cup of cheerios." I felt kind of stupid like I had just said,

"I carried a watermelon." But he didn't say anything so I didn't either but surely they will notice when I go next week. I was telling my sister about the diet again. Of course she wants to try it and is asking me a lot of questions about it. I thought today about how I am a human guinea pig, as no one has done this before and that is pretty exciting but at the same time what if it stopped. I would be very disappointed, but whose to say how long it will work. I guess all inventors have doubts. For lunch I had an awesome chicken salad sandwich. Food is so intense now. It tasted like a filet mignon. I am stuffed beyond belief. I only had one sandwich, toasted whole wheat bread, white chicken, and onion tomato with two tablespoons of regular mayonnaise. I am not eating any of that low fat diet crap again. My husband does all of our grocery shopping. Today he bought cookies and chips as always and I usually really complain about that because it is a lot easier to say no in the store than it is to say no at home. This time it doesn't bother me so much if I want a cookie I will eat one. A cookie is not going to own my whole life. Food is my bitch now, not the other way around.

I had a salmon patty, green beans and Mac and cheese for supper. It was amazing. Right now as I write this it is 2:14 a.m. on March 2, and I am still not hungry. Going to bed though cause I have my work finished.

Couldn't sleep, I am just so excited about this discovery. I read somewhere the other day where it said, "Americans need to change their eating habits." Well nothing could be further from the truth but not in the way most people think. Imagine this, walking into a restaurant and instead of seeing tables with multiple chairs you see feeding stations. Individual sectioned off centers where one person sits down and orders and eats.

The person would not be able to see or hear

anyone else in the restaurant. As any noise or distraction from eating will cause the diner to not be aware of what they are eating and they will continue to stay hungry. Families before have been encouraged to sit down at a family dinner each evening and talk about their day. This is the worst possible advice. Eating should never be an activity, and you should especially never mix it with conversation. Each family member should eat separately and quietly in space of their own. Radical ideas but I believe it will take something radical to change the obesity epidemic in our country. So many times at the dinner table instead of polite conversation, the conversation can be critical or stressful. This is the exact opposite of what mealtimes should be. I had a conversation with my sister where I explained the program to her. She is finding it hard to find a quiet time to eat. "Most of the time I grab a burrito and eat it going down the road," She said. This is going to be similar to a lot of people. I asked her, "If you pulled off the road, put in your earplugs and ate your burrito, how much time would you think that would take? Of course it would not take very long. I asked her if you drove down the road and you had to go to the bathroom what would you do? You would find a bathroom pull off to the side of the road and go to the bathroom. You would not wear a diaper, unless you had a medical condition. If you have time in your life to go to the bathroom by yourself, you should make time to eat by yourself. I know there will be women out there with young children that will proclaim they just don't have the time. I remember what it is like to have small children. If possible set an example to the children to eat quietly. I think it will be a good lifelong habit.

The rules for the Quiet Diet

There are not a lot of rules but they are very stringent. You cannot vary from them. I plan on writing a second book when I am closer to my goal weight and have developed the program more thoroughly. Here are rules so far.

1. Always, Always, Always wear earplugs when eating. Listen to every bite, chew, swish, and swallow. The internal sounds that your mouth makes in theory, is the reason your brain knows it has eaten. Once your brain hears you are eating, it will let you know when you are full. Respect the food by respecting the sanctity of eating.

2. Eat from a white eight-inch plate with no designs. If you do not have one, purchase one. Fill it once with the food you are going to eat for that meal. If you are still hungry you can always go back for more but it is doubtful you will be.

3. Eat three times a day. Never eat past 6 p.m.

4. Eat anything you want, if you want a cheeseburger start with half a cheeseburger or a small one, begin with small portions. Remember you can always go back for more.

5. Do not drink with your meal. You can have a drink available beside your plate in case you need to sip but drinks will cause you to "wash" the food down and that's not good.

6. Whenever possible eat at least one crunchy noisy food with your meal. The crunching, biting, chewing is your body's way of telling your brain that you have eaten. Eating is a sacred thing. I repeat, eating is a very sacred thing. If you must meet someone socially in a dining situation, always meet for coffee or drinks never meet them for a meal. Think of eating just as you would going to the bathroom. You would not meet friends in a communal toilet to talk while you all go to the bathroom. Do not meet them to eat either. Your meals should be spent quietly, head down eyes closed when chewing but you should open them to look at your food. You should breath out after each bite is swallowed and you will be able to tell you are full from eating when you start to sigh.

7. Try not to think about anything else but the food in your mouth when you are eating. Keep telling yourself mealtimes are sacred quiet times not to be interrupted.

I know the rule against dining out with friends will be met with negativity. First of all from restaurant owners but keep in mind there are plenty of skinny people out there that can still dine in restaurants. We, as fat people do not have that luxury until there is a restaurant with the foresight to set up a quiet diners booth for us to use much like the handicapped have their own bathroom. If your friends are going out to eat ask them what time, and show up after the meal for coffee.

March 2, 2011

I am not going to weigh until Monday when I will be past my period. Right after I explained the program to my sister, when we were getting ready to leave her house she said, 'Do you guys want to go to lunch, I will take you out to lunch." I said, "Remember that is like asking someone to go use the toilet with you, it's a no, no." I don't know if she gets it. On the bright side she gave me a whole bunch of her clothes she didn't want anymore and I can't wait until I can get into them. Some of them I can actually get in but they don't look good on me yet. I did find a really cute outfit that is a size 16 and I thought I might be able to wear that to my daughter's Graduation in May of next year. I did not overeat today or eat too much but I did have a little glass of orange juice tonight because I felt a little dehydrated that could be from my period. Sorry if you are a guy and are reading this, but we women have different issues when it comes to dieting.

March 3, 2011

Blood sugar 123 before meds, that's what I'm talkin' bout'! I only ate two meals today. I had two chicken salad sandwiches. I ate at 10 this morning and grew sleepy at about 12 p.m. after I had completed some work so I decided to lay down. When I awoke there was only time for one meal before 6 p.m. So now it is 8:30 p.m. and I am not sure if I should eat again or wait until tomorrow. Honestly I am not hungry. I think I will take my blood sugar. After eating all day my reading was 158 which is good I suppose since I use to have readings in the 300. I am dying to weigh but I promised myself I wouldn't weigh until Monday. My husband has been giving away some of our food to a bachelor neighbor since I am not eating as much. The other day when I made the salmon patties he had to give the leftovers away which was quite a bit. I cannot believe the massive amount of food I was ingesting.

I still have plenty of energy but because of my knee hurting I cannot do as much as I would like. I don't mean exercise, I hate exercise. I don't like to sweat if I can keep from it. Of course, like I have said before I am a human guinea pig and may have to exercise later but I will cross that bridge when I come to it.

March 4, 2011

Well I did it again, I messed up a little I had some popcorn last night. I am not weighing until Monday so I don't know if it affected my weight but my sugar this morning was 148 which is still really good for me, but I feel like it was the popcorn that made it jump. I didn't eat a lot of it but I was on my period and craving something salty and crunchy. I hate putting a lot of this personal information out in the public but if I am going to be a human guinea pig I feel I should be brutally honest. This morning for breakfast I had a cup of bran flakes and a slice of butter wheat toast. I tried to pay attention to my eating but I was upset when I was eating so I hope my brain still registers it as a meal. I will know later on if I am hungry. I was reading an article about consolidating all the small schools in our area and it really made me angry. Our small schools are the backbone of our community, and I hate to see them destroyed. I think of how hard our ancestors worked to get a school built in their community. It would be such a shame to lose them. Anyway, it really has nothing to do with the weight loss program but it is a good time to talk about stressors.

With this diet so far, I am on Day 9 and I have not reached a stressor that has made me binge yet, so that says something. I use to binge everyday.

I don't know if all binge eaters are like this but I hate to leave home. My husband does all the shopping. If I absolutely have to go somewhere I will. I also don't like to talk on the phone. I am hoping after I lose a bunch of weight that I will want to venture out more. There was a rumor going around that I had left my husband because no one in the neighborhood had seen me in so long. I don't have any real friends besides my family except online at social networking sites. I had an omelet for lunch, I made it with 3 eggs but could only eat half of it. I put in red peppers, bacon bits (real ones not imitation) and green onions it was so good. The flavors were so intense. I also had a glass of tomato juice. I am stuffed beyond belief. It's 4 p.m. and I will probably just eat a salad for supper.

I had a chicken and green beans with a glass of milk. I added a tablespoon of Barbeque sauce to the chicken. It was delicious. I am so amazed at the small portions I eat now.

March 5, 2011

Sugar 128 I am so excited. Even though I decided not to weigh until Monday. I am so happy about my low sugar readings if this keeps up I can see myself totally off my medication someday. (If my doctor agrees) I am going to the doctor on March 9 so I can ask him about all that then. The true test will come today. I have to take mother to the store for grocery shopping. If I can get in and out of her house and to the grocery store, without being forced fed, that will be a miracle.

Mission accomplished. When I picked her up the first thing she said was, "Now I am going to tell you something and don't get mad." To which I replied, "Okay but first I want to say something, 'You are not the boss of me" I said it in a very nice joking way but she got the message and during the entire trip every time she would try to feed me something I would just say, "No I don't want it" and then add, "Remember you are not the boss of me." Sure it sounds childish but when I am with my mother I am her child and however I can get through the day with out binge eating is okay. Another phrase I learned to use with my husband is to say, "I will have some if you will." He usually gets the point and quits trying to force it on me. I come from a long line of short fat women who suffered from the "disease to please." It is something I struggle with daily. You have to realize there is nothing wrong with putting yourself first.

In my research through books, articles and the net, statistics show approximately 60% of women are actively engaged in some kind of weight loss plan at any one moment in time. Unfortunately, studies show that only 5% of these weight loss plans and other solutions will ever do you any good as far as sustained weight loss goes. The reason the diets fail is because at some point the dieter, "goes off" the diet. With the "Quiet Diet" you could theoretically continue to wear the earplugs the rest of your life. You could continue eating anything you want.

March 6, 2011

Sugar 136

March 7, 2011

Well, I cannot lie, my weight today was 264. I wanted it to be more drastic but it wasn't. I am still sticking to the program, because well frankly, it is not that hard to do anyway. Today for breakfast I had half of a 3-egg omelet and toast and a half of an orange. For lunch I had 1 piece of pepperoni pizza and a garden salad. Yes, I know that sounds like a lot but it really was a very small piece and when I say garden salad, I mean lettuce, green onion, and carrot. Besides, I have always said you cannot stay on the diet unless you can eat foods you love. For supper I am having a chicken salad sandwich.

March 8, 2011

My weight is 260 today and sugar was 171. So happy about my weight I feel like I am back on track again. My sugar was too high but that is because I ate some popcorn before I went to bed. I have to stay away from the popcorn. I don't feel like it makes me gain weight but I feel like it raises my sugar too high.

I read two popular diet programs that said you could eat on the vegetables you want. Not sure if that is a good idea. I know that seems contradictory because I stated in this book you could eat all you want, but keep in mind with this program you won't "want". So eating a massive amount of veggies is really not an option. I am not sure allowing a binge eater to eat all they want of one thing is a good idea.

Tomorrow I will weigh again and I am excited about that. I am also excited to see my doctor and ask him what he thinks of my diet. I am not going to tell him about the earplugs only about the amount of food I am eating. I think he is going to be pleased about my sugar readings. I have no way to check my blood pressure so that will be interesting to find out as well.
Tomorrow at 3 p.m. I will visit my doctor and weigh in. I am not going to tell him about the

program yet. I do have some questions about my Diabetes though.

Great doctor's appointment, I left there very happy! He said whatever you are doing keep doing it. He also said if I am still losing in May he would redo my blood work and if was okay he would see about taking me off my diabetes medicine. He said he was very proud of me. I had to laugh at that one. What is there to be proud of? I have been eating pizza, spaghetti, whatever I like, it has not been like I am suffering.

I was sad to hear the discoloration in my feet and legs will not go away even if I lose weight. I wish I had not gained so much weight but I refuse to look back with regret. What is that saying, "The more you know, the better you do." I know better now. He didn't mention exercise and neither did I. I know exercise is good for you, but I have mixed feelings about it. When I was around 35 years old I got what I can only describe as a "rush of hormones." I began excercising like crazy. I would walk two miles a day, one mile on a circle track and one mile on a hiking trail. I was also swimming three times a week. Keep in mind I was still binge eating so I wasn't small, I was packing a lot of weight around and that was the beginning of my knee injury. I know if there is a skinny person reading this, they are skeptical. Any excuse not to exercise huh? Well, I just don't like exercise and I especially don't like it when it is painful. There may come a day on this journey when I do have to up my physical activity and when that day comes I will do what I need to do to try and lose weight but I won't be happy about it.

I do not want to tell people what to eat. That may sound crazy since this is a diet book. However I feel there is no way I could design a diet that would fit everyone's lifestyle and cultural differences. Living in a Native American community and rural area, sometimes my family eats squirrel, deer, catfish, and wild onions. I couldn't imagine leaving those things out of my diet but I doubt any of those foods are listed in popular diet books. My advice for anyone who wants to lose weight is to eat what you normally eat but in smaller portions. That doesn't mean cheese puffs for every meal. There are plenty of menus out there from the government nutritional websites, which are totally free. If you wear the earplugs, use the plate and follow the recommendations in the book you should do just fine. I would advise this. Eat what you like, if there is an opportunity to cook it in a more healthy way then that is ideal. I don't believe in giving up the things you love. I have eaten chili pies, spaghetti, pizza etc. since I started this diet. Like I said if I want a cookie I will eat a cookie. It really doesn't matter what you eat because you will not be able to eat very much anyway.

What This Diet Can Do For You

There is a popular quote that says, "The definition of insanity is doing the same thing over and over and expecting different results." Let's face it folks, we have all tried the "Diet and Exercise" myth for years and it is not working. If it were working obesity rates would not be as high as they are now. It's time to make some radical changes in the way we eat and the way we serve our food.

If you want a diet where you can eat anything you want, as much as you want, with no exercise. This is the diet for you. There are no powders, pills, formulas, points or packaged foods for you to buy. I believe with my whole heart and with all the best intentions that this program will help you lose weight.

There are people out there who want you to believe that every fat person is fat because of emotional eating. In my humble opinion there is no such thing. That to me is a stereotype, they see fat people as being fat with a bundle of nerves, either crying at the drop of a hat over their problems or being jolly. I will be so bold as to say fat people are not over emotional. They are fat because they don't know how to switch their brain off and tell their stomach that they are full. A fat person's emotions are no different from a skinny person. There is nothing innate that says that a skinny person is more mentally healthy than a fat person. To me that is just a myth. I also think it is something fat people have known all along. If you only have 5-20 pounds to lose, I do not know if this diet work.

I know this program has helped me. I was binge eater, consuming massive amounts of food, in secret. My hope is that this book will generate new interest and open the door to debate on this issue. I am hoping this will stimulate new research in the search for a cure for obesity. For some it may raise a lot of questions. For me, it is the answer I have searched for my whole life and I thank God I found it.

Since starting this program, I keep telling everyone in my family, this must be what it feels like to be normal, to be that woman that only eats a half of a sandwich or to not have food control your every entire waking moment

This book may seem haphazard, if so, I apologize. I have to get the information out there. People are dying from obesity and if this is a cure, people need to know. We must begin the conversation. We must start the debate. We must let people know that they don't have to suffer any longer.

What does the future hold for me? Will I continue to lose weight? Will I hit a dieting plateau and have to begin an exercise program? I don't know the answer to these questions. I cannot even tell you why the program works but it works for me.

I hope it will help you too.